A BLUEPRINT FOR HEALTHY EATING:

YOUR DIET GUIDE FOR THE NEW

MILLENNIUM

Nicholas H.E. Mezitis, M.D.

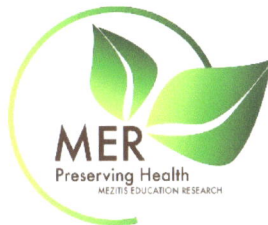

MER
Preserving Health
MEZITIS EDUCATION RESEARCH

First Printing: 2017

ISBN 978-0692294284

Mezitis Education Research, LLC

PO Box 741

Athens, OH 45701

This book is dedicated in loving memory to my parents,

Elias and Sophia, with gratitude.

About the Author

Dr. Nicholas H.E. Mezitis trained in Endocrinology and Nutrition at St. Luke's/Roosevelt Hospital Center of Columbia University College of Physicians and Surgeons and at the Memorial Sloan-Kettering Cancer Center. He was a Fellow in Diabetes and Endocrinology at the Joslin Diabetes Center – Harvard University and the New England Deaconess Hospital. He served residencies in Internal Medicine at Thomas Jefferson University Hospital in Philadelphia and in Clinical and Anatomic Pathology at the George Washington University Hospital in Washington, D.C. He is a graduate of the Ruprecht Karl University Medical School in Heidelberg, Germany, where he was awarded his doctoral title 'Magna Cum Laude'.

Dr. Mezitis is Associate Professor of Specialty Medicine at Ohio University Heritage College of Osteopathic Medicine. He has been active in research since 1985, participating in clinical trials investigating many of the important new medications currently in use for the management of diabetes mellitus, obesity, and osteoporosis. He is the recipient of numerous research grants and he helped create and direct the Clinical Pharmacology Program at St. Luke's/Roosevelt Hospital Center for pharmaceutical research.

Dr. Mezitis' special area of interest is clinical nutrition and metabolism. He has taught Nutrition to physicians in the Fellowship Program at St. Luke's/ Roosevelt Hospital Center and to dieticians at Columbia University Teachers College. He is a lecturer at the Columbia University Masters Program in Nutrition. Nutrition is the foundation of patient management in his clinical practice.

Acknowledgments

I am deeply appreciative of the insights imparted by my mentors Dr. Sami Hashim and Dr. F. Xavier Pi-Sunyer over many years of association at the Obesity Research Center of St. Luke's/Roosevelt Hospital Center / Columbia University in New York. I also wish to thank Heidi Mochari, R.D. who worked on materials provided in the Appendices to complement the text. Samuel Wagner, medical student, assisted in the design and graphics in this work and I sincerely appreciate his collaboration.

The Blueprint itself reflects the Hippocratic ideal of 'Πὰν μέτρον ἄριστον' ('All in good measure') and the precept of inclusion and balance, rather than exclusion and vilification of food choices. Any shortcomings on the presentation of material in this diet guide are my responsibility.

TABLE OF CONTENTS

1
FOREWORD

Nutrition is established as the cornerstone of health. Protein, fat, carbohydrate, vitamins, minerals, and water are the building blocks for our bodies and the fuel for our activities. Simple as it may appear, our separation as an urbanized society from the sources of our food has added complexity to planning nutritious meals on a daily basis. Much of what is available to us on store shelves and in eating establishments offers many calories, but little nutritional value, not to speak of hazards posed by additives to the food supply. More importantly, the facility with which these calories can be obtained, involving minimal physical activity on our part, creates an energy imbalance from the first bite. As if this were not enough, advertising and peer pressure promote an imbalance on our plate dominated by simple sugars and sweeteners married with oil blends, in their many guises.

I have been fortunate to have been exposed to the 'farm to fork' traditional culture during my formative years and to have appreciated the exquisite variety of flavors that nature provides us with in abundance. In medical school, it became clear to me that complex biochemistry and pathophysiology was really very simple in its message when translated to the reality of our meal. In my postgraduate training, I benefited from mentors who are pioneers in the field of nutrition and metabolism and who helped me distill my knowledge on these topics into a lucid message for my patients.

It is this message that I wish to impart in my book. A message that I deliver daily to my patients struggling with a wide variety of health issues: if the fuel mix is neglected and deliveries are chaotic, addressing symptoms and signs of illness becomes inconsequential.

A Blueprint for Healthy Eating: Your Diet Guide for the New Millennium should help you understand the reason for balance on the meal plate and rhythm in the timing of meals. If it achieves this goal, it is a mission completed. In the words of Hippocrates: Our food should be our medicine and our medicine should be our food.

2

INTRODUCTION

"There's only one diet."

The purpose of my book is to provide a *guide for the eating experience* in our modern multiethnic society, where calories are inexpensive and foods are available in endless variety. The body does not come with an instruction manual, yet precisely such a set of guidelines appears to be necessary for our diet, which plays a critical role in defining health.

In all major cities, we are surrounded by food available in settings ranging from the supermarket and the corner grocery to fast food outlets, ethnic restaurants, and fine culinary establishments. Chefs enjoy superstar status. Cooking courses abound. Meals can be delivered directly to the home or workplace at all hours, throughout the year.

TV and radio have no shortage of talk shows and sound bites addressing diet-related topics. Bookstores are filled with titles on food preparation and diet recommendations. Hundreds of articles are published every year in scientific journals presenting the results of studies relating to nutrition and health. Magazines feature the message of the day, reviewing the do's and don'ts of eating in every issue.

Confronted with such a flood of information and such a boundless array of choices, the experience for many of us can be that of a boat adrift in high seas. Traditional diets are being challenged. Familiar foods are being associated with major health problems. Culinary pleasures have become threats for reasons unclear.

A blueprint sets the stage for building and my book strives to do the same for the diet experience. It is not intended to replace the literature available, but rather to guide the reader in making the best use of available resources. As such, it explains the relationships between varying dietary trends and it suggests choices, which contribute to a healthy and productive life.

Health and the pleasure derived from enjoying a well prepared, appealing meal are not incompatible. Quite the contrary, a *meal must be enjoyed* in order for the body to derive maximum nutritional value from the experience. The reader will become an informed consumer using the wide variety of available food choices and diet resources in a responsible manner, to derive benefit and minimize health risks.

3

DIGESTION & METABOLISM
"You are what you eat."

'A magical mystery tour'
Our body composition reflects the content of our diet. All foods, whether of animal or vegetable origin, are made up of protein, carbohydrate and fat with water, vitamins and minerals in varying proportions. Consumed as part of a meal, foods undergo a transformation process in the body. First, they are broken down to their basic components in the intestine. This means that protein will be digested to amino acids, fat to fatty acids and triglycerides, and carbohydrate to monosaccharides. Only these simple nutrient building blocks, along with vitamins, minerals and water, can be absorbed by the gut. Traveling rapidly through the lymphatics and the bloodstream these vital materials reach the liver. There, cellular machinery uses them to create our own special proteins and fat. Sugar is used as fuel for this and other activities and the excess is stored in liver and muscle as glycogen or in adipose tissue as fat. Food has now been transformed into our own image and we have been transformed by our food.

The mouth – 'Unwrapping the meal'
Digestion begins in the mouth, where the teeth grind down dietary grains, vegetables and animal tissues. The tongue mixes carbohydrates, proteins and fats with saliva and the breakdown of starch to simple sugars begins. Nature's packaging for starch is cellulose, which represents the fiber in our diet. Cellulose cannot

15

be absorbed by our digestive system. Once it has been ruptured by the teeth and vigorously ground in the stomach, its water, minerals and starch content are extracted in the intestine. Residual cellulose fibers form the bulk of the stool, trapping water, distending the bowel and stimulating its movement.

The stomach – 'The blender'

Food materials we swallow are gently pushed through the esophagus and land in a pool of acid in the stomach, released in anticipation of their arrival. The acid denatures protein, destroying bacteria and other life forms before they can gain access to the lush, absorptive surface of the intestine. The stomach with its slimy lining, covered with chemically active secretions, grinds and mixes the foods, preparing them for gradual release into the small intestine through a special exit, the pylorus. The speed with which the stomach empties its contents is influenced by the amount of fat in the foods it is processing.

The small intestine – 'Absorbing the meal'

In the small intestine, the residual stomach acid mixed with the food is neutralized. Only then can the bile and the pancreatic juices, which contain enzymes that require an alkaline environment, begin their work. Lipase, one of the pancreatic enzymes, digests the fat in the food. Bile released from the gallbladder covers the products of fat digestion, making them water-soluble so the intestine can absorb them. Two other pancreatic enzymes, trypsin and amylase complete the digestion of protein. Amino acids, the valuable building blocks of protein, can now be absorbed, without the risk of foreign life forms entering our system. Vitamins and minerals follow the flow, linking up with other food ingredients or intestinal factors to make the trip across the intestinal wall into the lymphatics and the bloodstream.

Lymphocytes – 'Immigration'

Monitoring this flurry of activity on the intestinal carpet is the body's defense force, the lymphocytes. Some are conveniently clustered in observation posts ('tonsils') bulging from the intestinal wall into its lumen. Others circulate freely in the blood stream and the lymph bathing the intestine, while many are patiently stationed in lymph node filters on the other side of the intestinal wall, examining the nutrients, which are absorbed. From their various vantage points the lymphocytes scan the incessant traffic entering the lymphatic highway from the intestine on its way to our blood stream for distribution throughout the body. They are our 'immigration service', identifying and sometimes tagging useful nutrients for future reference, while remaining vigilant for dangerous substances and life forms. Amino acids, glucose and fatty acids travel this pathway into the blood steam and on to the liver, our factory where chemical processing and production lines never stop.

The liver – 'Bank and factory'

Glucose sugar is the life fuel on which the brain depends. Fluctuations in glucose supply can lead to dangerous 'brownouts' for the nervous system, which we know as 'hypoglycemia'. Hypoglycemia can lead to data processing errors, confusion and even death, just as surely as a computer's hard drive can be irreparably damaged by electrical power fluctuations. The liver's primary assignment is to be a glucose 'bank', storing this valuable fuel so that it can be rapidly available to the system, in case of delays in meal deliveries. If fasting is prolonged, the liver can also transform fat and protein into glucose, in order to replenish supplies. Such a superb performance enables the body to maintain blood glucose levels stable within a very narrow range at all times.

The liver also functions as a powerful 'factory.' Its busy cells receive amino acids and fatty acids from the intestine after every meal. They create protein, which the body needs to grow, function and move. They make fat, which lubricates and insulates the body's tissues and provides energy storage capacity.

Insulin – 'The playmaker'

Insulin is the key to the liver's activities. First, it promotes the entry of glucose into liver cells. Then, it ensures that the glucose absorbed by the cells is stored as glycogen, rather than consumed to fuel other activities. Likewise, insulin promotes fat and protein creation from fatty acids and amino acids, respectively, resulting in weight gain and muscle growth. Vitamins and minerals participate in this 'festival of growth', either as regulators of the activities or as essential building blocks themselves.

But insulin is not the body's growth hormone simply because of its effect on the liver. Nutrients from the meal need to enter cells throughout the body and to be utilized immediately or stored. Insulin exerts its regulatory role everywhere in the body. Key 'target tissues' for insulin, however, are fat and muscle. Insulin again is the playmaker, facilitating the entry of nutrients into cells and defining their disposition as glycogen or fat stores or as protein. 'Thrift' is the name of the game for this important player.

Fasting – 'Tapping into savings'

When the body fasts for short periods, such as when we sleep overnight, nutrient absorption slacks off and insulin levels drop. The liver, relieved slightly from its demanding supervisor, loses its motivation to keep glucose in storage. It begins to break down its glycogen stores releasing glucose into the bloodstream to maintain circulating levels in a steady range. The same events take place in muscle as fasting continues.

Longer periods of fasting fully deplete glycogen stores in the liver and in the muscle. After roughly 24 hours, fat and protein stores in adipose tissue and muscle are mobilized to obtain ingredients for glucose production. Fat meltdown also produces acid in the form of ketones. These substances can themselves serve as rapidly available fuel both for the brain and for other tissues, providing insulin is available to regulate traffic.

The contra-insulin hormones – 'The linebackers'
When we fast, several other important hormones declare themselves as defenders of our glucose supply. They single-mindedly oppose insulin action in order to ensure plentiful supplies of fat and protein for glucose production by the liver. These are the 'contra-insulin hormones': cortisol, epinephrine, nor-epinephrine, glucagon, and growth hormone being the most important. Their role is to ensure an adequate supply of the brain's preferred fuel, glucose, at all costs. Tissue meltdown is the result.

Insulin and contra-insulin hormones in balance – 'a metabolic melody'

The balance of insulin, glucose and contra-insulin hormones is a delicate one. When properly functioning, it results in a finely regulated level of glucose in the blood. Wild swings in blood glucose level, either into the high (hyperglycemia) or low (hypoglycemia) ranges are prevented. To achieve this, the body's fuel sensor - the pancreatic beta cell – must finely tune its insulin release to match meal requirements. Alerted to insulin's activities, the other hormones follow suit, harmoniously balancing its effects.

For the individual, the key to maintaining the smooth metabolic rhythm described is to 'tread gently' with balanced meals, properly timed and consumed in a relaxed environment with particular focus on proper food preparation and patient chewing.

A diet prescription is urgently required.

4

DIET PRINCIPLES
"Everything in moderation"

Which is the diet for me? – 'Confusion vs. simplicity'
There is only one healthy diet for any given population group.
This point has been obscured by the glut of information relating
to food, which has flooded television, radio, the print media, and
more recently the electronic media. Much of what we say will
apply to populations residing in the temperate zones of the planet,
such as the United States.

Over the past decade in the United States, we have seen the
introduction of low fat - high carbohydrate Asian cuisine and its
varied permutations. We have witnessed the wide acceptance of
the moderate fat 'Mediterranean diet', rich in olive oil. We have
read reports of the "French paradox" with red wine
complementing foie gras in promoting longevity. We have heard
of the benefits of yogurt consumed by centenarians in Armenia
and of Umeboshi plums savored by their gracefully aging
counterparts in Okinawa. The food pyramid has replaced the food
wheel and we may yet witness the 'food cube' or some other
geometric construct.

The public's attention has been focused on seeking out the
differences in these diet approaches, in the hope of identifying the
unique diet modification ensuring life and health everlasting. This
approach is non-productive. I suggest we *seek out the existing
similarities*, which will serve the same purpose much more

effectively. In doing so, we must not lose sight of the fact that the human digestive system is delicately designed to make use of a wide variety of food sources. It is this property that characterizes us as 'omnivorous'. Being selective in our food choices is appropriate however, since population groups acclimatized to their traditional habitats and local food sources over millennia. Likewise, the seasonal change in the food supply according to geographic region is not without reason.

Dietary balance – 'Variety is the key'

Contemplating the above, note that Nature in her wisdom provides all the nutrients we require in forms that permit balance in the diet and promote satiety, while preserving smooth digestive function. Vegetables are the most abundant food source and provide starch, fiber, water, oils, minerals and vitamins. Seasonal variation ensures a balanced presentation of a variety of the above ingredients to the body over the course of a calendar year. Grains require cultivation and processing, but also offer an excellent source of carbohydrate and minerals. Fruits enhance the diet with their taste, while delivering water, carbohydrate, minerals, vitamins, and in some instances oils. The flesh of mammals, fish, and poultry as well as their products in the form of dairy, eggs, and oils provide valuable protein and essential fat to replenish and fuel the body's tissues. Legumes (beans) have a similar role to play.

The proportions of different foods in the diet and their most appropriate preparation for the meal have been the subject of ongoing debate. Here again we should take our cues from Nature herself. Vegetables, as mentioned, are provided in greatest abundance and should form the foundation of the diet. A representation of 40% of daily calories from this source is not excessive. Grains have their vital role to play and minimally processed should deliver another 20% of the daily calorie allowance, at least. Fat adds flavor to the meal apart from its nutrient value and should be considered for not more than 30% of calories, while valuable protein should make up for the balance. Expressed in grams, the amount of protein on a daily basis generally should not exceed 1 g for each kg of a healthy person's body weight.

Food choices – 'From prescription to the kitchen'
The type of protein, fat and carbohydrate to be selected has also been the topic of heated debate. Here we should take into account factors such as the traditional habitat of population groups, medical illnesses, physical limitations and diet preferences. Vegetables and grains again deserve to be heavily represented as sources of carbohydrate and oil, while legumes should not be neglected as a complementary protein source. Variety is key in stimulating all parts of the digestive system and in ensuring an adequate supply of vitamins, trace elements and minerals for the body.

The processing and storage of foods are key issues for consideration as we make our choices at the market. Fresh is best. There is no question that the nutritional adequacy of foods diminishes as their final consumption is delayed. Fortunately, technology not only permits fortification of foods with vitamins and minerals lost in processing, but it is also in position to restrict degradation of nutrients by interfering with bacterial and fungal proliferation. These advances have enabled vast segments of the world population to enjoy vital diet options previously restricted to a privileged few. Prolongation of the human life span is in large part due to better nutrition.

The source of our food is very important. It is said that the ancient Greeks, in deciding on the most appropriate location for a new city, would visit the site under consideration in the spring and release a cow for pasture. If the animal was still alive after the winter, this was taken to be proof of adequate food resources in the vicinity and mitigated in the site's favor. The animal was then sacrificed and its liver was carefully examined. A healthy liver was considered to reflect a healthy environment, fit for human settlement. Accordingly, not only an adequate food supply, but also a quality food supply is of paramount importance as we select our food.

The chemical industry has enabled agricultural wonders to be realized on a global scale, feeding millions and contributing greatly to the population boom. On an individual basis, as we confront acute and chronic illness, the price of some of this technology becomes a growing issue of concern. Pesticides, antibiotics, hormonal and protein supplements are now pervasive in the food supply and their accumulation in our bodies is a reality. The health implications of this development cannot be ignored. Both allergies and infectious diseases have been associated with this type of dietary intervention.

Irradiation of foods also raises important issues relating to changes in vital nutrients and how they affect our body. Genetic manipulation of the food supply is the latest arrival on the food-processing scene and again technology is far ahead of our understanding of the risk: benefit ratio for consumers.

Meal preparation – 'From the kitchen to the plate'

A word of introduction on meal preparation is now appropriate. Foods should be properly cleansed, lightly seasoned as per preference and gently cooked where appropriate. Cooking of protein, particularly that of animal origin, is of course very appropriate, considering the realities of our modern food supply, where contamination with forms of life noxious for humans is becoming increasingly prevalent. Vegetables and fruits on the other hand should be consumed fresh, if possible, taking into consideration local factors which would dictate special cleansing or peeling of skins or even light cooking. Oils and butters should also be enjoyed fresh. Heating of fats to high temperatures generates chemicals such as acroleins, which may irritate and damage the digestive system.

Dietary goals – 'Maintaining vigor'

If our goal is to age gracefully and to minimize our contacts with physicians to social events, an apple a day will no longer suffice. The chemical exposures of the apple and of the tree and of the entire food supply must be considered. Visually perfect produce is not the goal. Rather, we should strive for nutritious produce with minimal chemical contamination bearing the minor blemishes, which are nature's quality seals of approval. Produce not fit for a fungus to grow on can certainly not be expected to optimally support human growth and fitness.

Summary – 'Our plan'

In summary, when the choice is available, food should be seasonal, fresh and in its most natural form. Meal preparation should be expedited, minimizing the need for prolonged food storage. Food preparation for meals should be gentle and simple, with limited heating and processing. The amount of food prepared should not be excessive, so that each meal may be a fresh one.

This approach enables us to derive the highest nutritional value from each meal, since the degradation process for macronutrients (starch, protein, fat) and for micronutrients such as vitamins begins at harvest time and is accelerated through cooking. It also preserves the unique flavors of the various ingredients making the eating experience a true pleasure.

5

THE DIET PRESCRIPTION
"Your personal food label"

Body Composition – 'The virtual label'
We are all familiar with the labels on food packages listing ingredients in detail (Fig. 5.1). The labels also provide information on calories per serving and the breakdown of each serving in terms of fat, protein, carbohydrate and electrolytes such as sodium and potassium. Vitamin content is also listed.

Our body carries a similar 'virtual' label (Fig. 5.2). We see that most of our makeup is water, which we primarily carry packaged inside our billions of cell packages. Smaller amounts of water circulate in our blood vessels and lymphatics and an even smaller amount bathes our cells as they are suspended in the various tissues. Water can be circulated and stored in this fashion because cells and vessels all become water-tight by a thin covering of fat, which the body can selectively manipulate to allow for transfer of fat and nutrients.

Fig. 5.1

Nutrition Facts

21 servings per container

Serving size   **2 crackers (14g)**

Amount Per Serving

Calories   60

	% Daily Value*
Total Fat 1.5g	**2%**
Saturated Fat 0g	**0%**
Trans Fat 0g	
Cholesterol 0mg	**0%**
Sodium 70mg	**3%**
Total Carbohydrate 10g	**4%**
Dietary Fiber 1g	**4%**
Total Sugars 0g	
Includes 0g Added Sugars	**0%**
Protein 2g	**4%**
Vitamin D 0mcg	0%
Calcium 0mg	0%
Iron 0.36mg	2%
Potassium 0mg	0%

*The % Daily Value (DV) tells you how much a nutrient in a serving of food contributes to a daily diet. 2,000 calories a day is used for general nutrition advice.

Fig. 5.2

Nutrition Facts
Human Body

Total Caloric Content

Calories   154,760

Body Composition (73kg Body Weight)	%
Water 45 kg	62%
Total Fat 11.7 kg	16%
Trans Fat 0 g	
Cholesterol 38 g	
Total Mineral	6%
Total Carbohydrate 11.7 kg	1%
Protein 11.7 kg	16%
Sodium	0.2%
Potassium	0.4%
Calcium 1.1 kg	1.5%
Iron	0.005%

Ingredients (Elemental): Oxygen, Carbon, Hydrogen, Nitrogen, Calcium, Phosphorus, Potassium, Sulphur, Sodium, Chlorine, Magnesium, Other

Macronutrients and Micronutrients – *'Nature's building blocks'*

Protein is the building material of life. It forms muscle, which permits movement. It forms the communications substrate in the brain and vital hormones that regulate our fuel management or metabolism. Fat stores energy, insulates nerves and protects cell contents. Carbohydrates provide energy for immediate use. Calcium and the other minerals give us a firm structure to suspend our tissues and, together with the vitamins, permit the chemical processes of life to proceed smoothly.

In planning our meal, we consider providing all of the required ingredients on our 'label': water, protein, fat, carbohydrate, vitamins and minerals. The amounts depend on our size, age and gender with consideration for our level of physical activity.

Counting Calories – ''Savings and checking'

The currency we deal with in balancing our metabolic 'check book' is the calorie. It represents a specific amount of energy to be generated by burning a specific dietary ingredient. For example, burning 1 gram of fat will generate 9 calories of energy, while burning 1 gram of protein generates only 4 calories (Fig.). It quickly becomes obvious why the body prefers to store energy in the form of fat, instead of carbohydrate or protein ('more mileage to the gallon').

When we plan our diet, the first thing we calculate is the caloric 'allowance'. This relates to our height, age, gender, and level of physical activity, as stated. The formula we use relates our daily energy requirement at rest (otherwise known as resting metabolic rate or daily energy expenditure) to our activity requirements. The calculation we make uses desirable body weight for a given height as a starting point. The calorie allowance calculated will permit weight maintenance for those individuals at target weight, while guiding the overweight to shed pounds and the underweight to add pounds. (Table 3).

[Height in cm (inches x 2.54) - 100] x 0.9 = desirable body weight (kilograms)

Desirable body weight (kg) x 24 = daily energy requirement at rest (calories)

The daily energy requirement is increased by 30% for average physical activity, 50% for moderate sports activity and it is doubled for individuals with a strenuous athletic program.

Protein in the diet is calculated generously to provide an average 1 g per kg (2.2 lbs) body weight. That would represent roughly 70 g for most people, translating into 210 calories (70 g x 4cal/g), to be subtracted from our allowance.

The remainder of the calorie allowance is divided between fat and carbohydrate. Fat should not exceed 30% of non-protein calories. The balance goes to carbohydrate.

Minerals and Vitamins

Calcium is a critical mineral for the body since it is so important in stabilizing the skeleton and in permitting all muscular activity. Modern diets with their emphasis on dairy restriction because of concerns about weight and atherosclerosis do not provide the necessary daily requirement to replace losses and to permit bone renewal to proceed. As people live longer and their bone structure weakens, we now have an osteoporosis epidemic looming. Calcium intake must be secured, if not as food choices, then at least in supplement form.

Sodium, on the other hand, is abundantly available in the diet of industrialized societies. A far cry from the time of ancient Rome when legionnaires received a salt allotment as payment for services ('salary'), we are now awash in dietary salt as a quick scan of supermarket food labels will reveal to the casual observer. This excess salt in a population that rarely sweats, due to lack of physical activity, poses a huge burden on the kidney to dispose of. Water retention and even an increase in blood pressure frequently result. Moderation is imperative and a 4 g allowance is both generous and realistic.

The other minerals and the vitamins are readily available when food choices and food preparation are planned as noted in our chapter on Diet Principles. Some individuals, particularly the elderly and those with chronic illnesses such as diabetes, may require vitamin and mineral supplements, since the diet may not meet their needs for various reasons. Those considerations are best planned in association with the physician and the dietitian.

Examples of Diet Prescription:
For the majority of the population, the following examples serve to illustrate our approach:

Table 5.1

Example 1:
40 y.o. moderately active, healthy female 5'6", 135 lbs (61 kg)
Calorie allowance: 2100 calories
Protein: 61 g or 244 calories
Non-protein calories: 1856 calories
Fat: 557 calories (0.30 x 1856) or 62 g (557/9)
Carbohydrate: 1299 calories (1856 – 557) or 325 g (1299/4)
Water: 7-8-glasses/ day
Sodium: 4 g
Calcium: 1500 mg
Vitamins: RDA

Table 5.2

Example 2:
28-year-old athletic male, 6', 183 lbs (76 kg)
Calorie allowance: 3580 calories
Protein: 76g or 304 calories
Non-protein calories: 3276 calories
Fat: 983 calories (0.30 x 3276) or 110 g (983/9)
Carbohydrate: 2293 calories (3276 - 983) or 574 g (2293/4)
Water: 16 glasses/day
Sodium: 6 g
Calcium: 1500 mg
Vitamins: RDA

Table 5.3

Example 3:
60-year-old female, limited activity due to arthritis in the knees, 5'4", 130 lbs
Calorie allowance: 1600 calories
Protein: 60 g or 240 calories
Non-protein calories: 1360 calories
Fat: 408 calories (1360 x 0.30) or 45 g (408/9)
Carbohydrate: 952 calories (1360 – 408) or 238 g (952/4)
Water: 6-8 glasses/day
Sodium: 2 g
Calcium: 1000 mg
Vitamins: RDA

(Note: The calorie allowance in the third example is based on the desirable body weight as usual. It is not based on the individual's actual weight and it should therefore help generate a 'calorie deficit' to promote weight reduction and hopefully alleviate the knee pain.)

Using these examples calculate your own 'prescription'.

Your diet prescription:

Calories	
Protein	
Fat	
Carbohydrate Water	
Calcium	
Sodium 4 g.	

6

FOOD SHOPPING
"Your food compass"

'The Perfect Storm'
Entering a modern food mega store can provide the white-knuckle experience of the Andrea Gail steaming into the eye of the 'mother of all storms.' Gleaming aisles with endless arrays of sparkling cans and colorful boxes stacked to the rafters assault the senses with conflicting colors and scents. Soothing images associated with 'mother, America, and apple pie' beckon the consumer. Music unravels the mind, interrupted by announcements of sales and 'specials.' Chilling temperatures in the periphery of the stores push the escaping customer back into the illusory comfort of the aisles … where the sales waves crest.

In order to weather the storm and successfully emerge with the 'catch,' the consumer-skipper needs education. The four basic tenets for food shopping are:

- **Be prepared**
- **Be focused**
- **Be picky**
- **And be quick.**

Shopping Lists - 'Be prepared'

Choices in the supermarket are endless and the prepared consumer finds that lists direct him swiftly to the items required. The staples of the diet -dairy, eggs, produce, meats, poultry, and fish - are all arrayed in the periphery of the store, usually requiring a long circumferential walk. The aisles have boxed, canned and bottled goods, which are the product of food processing. Most of our problems relating to dietary issues concern items stocked in the aisles, so the faster we complete this part of our selections the better. Inappropriate food choices stocked in the home virtually guarantee deviations from the meal plan.

The Diet Prescription – 'Be focused'

The shopper should always remember their diet prescription (Chapter 5) as they work their way through the store making selections. The items should preferably be fresh. Extraneous 'comfort foods' and snacks should be avoided. These are generally rich in sugars, salt and saturated oils. Interestingly, many such items are stocked near the checkout counters, presenting a special challenge to self-discipline for shoppers and their children waiting patiently in line.

The Food Labels – 'Be picky'

Food labels (Chapter 5) are valuable guides in making choices. Salt content and fat composition are important considerations. Foods containing hydrogenated fats and coconut oils are best avoided. Sugar as the first ingredient listed on the food label denotes a problem item with a high *glycemic index*. The latter is a measure of the blood sugar response to a particular food, with a greater spike in blood sugar following the consumption of foods rich in simple sugars. Foods grown without the use of pesticides, antibiotics and chemical fertilizers pose less of a burden for our body and should be preferred, if available. Foods and beverages in glass containers and paper boxes tend to react less with the container and are generally preferable to those packaged in plastic containers and metal cans. Quality is always a better value for our money as compared to quantity, even if it means eating less of a particular item.

Food Stores are for Food Shopping – 'Be quick'
Supermarkets invite browsing, lingering, and even socializing, which prolongs the consumers' exposure to the choices offered. Invariably, these delays result in selections unrelated to the required items with less concern for the diet prescription. The best approach is to use the list, shop the periphery of the store, quickly traverse the aisles and head for the cashier.

7

FOOD PREPARATION
"Nutritious can be delicious"

Culinary Education
Culinary literacy is a goal to be realized for our population.
Increasingly, we have become alienated from our food supply as
fewer people have direct contact with growing of crops and
flowers. Even more worrisome is the ignorance most people have
of basic food preparation. The fractured family with grandparents,
parents and children all pursuing separate activities has interfered
with the transfer of important knowledge and skills relating to
food selection and meal preparation.

Food Handling and Cooking
Foods should be purchased fresh, whenever possible and their
preservation in refrigeration should be minimized. Most foods,
including meats, should be washed with cold running water before
we proceed with meal preparation. Fresh salads provide valuable
vitamins, fiber and water and should be chewed thoroughly to
access the nutrients. Vegetables can also be sliced to disrupt cell
structures and permit cooking and digestive juices to access the
cell contents. Light steaming or braising should be sufficient for
vegetables requiring cooking. These processes enhance
digestibility while avoiding destruction of vitamins in the foods.
Olive oil, lemon juice, balsamic vinegar with salt or oregano serve
to enhance taste.

Whole grain products, short grain brown rice, and pasta are represented on the plate in small amounts (1 cup/meal). Beans and egg whites can be valuable protein sources and should be incorporated into the diet on a frequent basis. Meat and poultry require thorough cooking, while fish can be lightly broiled or grilled. Fresh or dried fruit, nuts and honey provide tasty dessert options. Herbal teas and sparkling or regular water are all we need to meet our fluid requirements.

The plate (Fig. 7.1 & 7.2) should include representatives of all the foods mentioned with an emphasis on vegetables and protein. Whole grains, brown rice, legumes, and fruits complete the picture.

BREAKFAST

Olive Oil
Canola Oil

Lean Meat
Egg White
Cheese
Yogurt

Olive Oil
Canola Oil
Tahini

Protein

Fruit

Grains/Starch

Milk
Herbal Tea
Water

Melon
Berries
Banana
Orange
Grapefruit
Apricots
Dates
Pineapple

Bread
Cereal
Oatmeal
Crackers
Pancakes

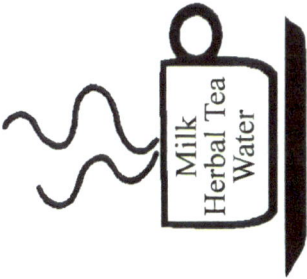

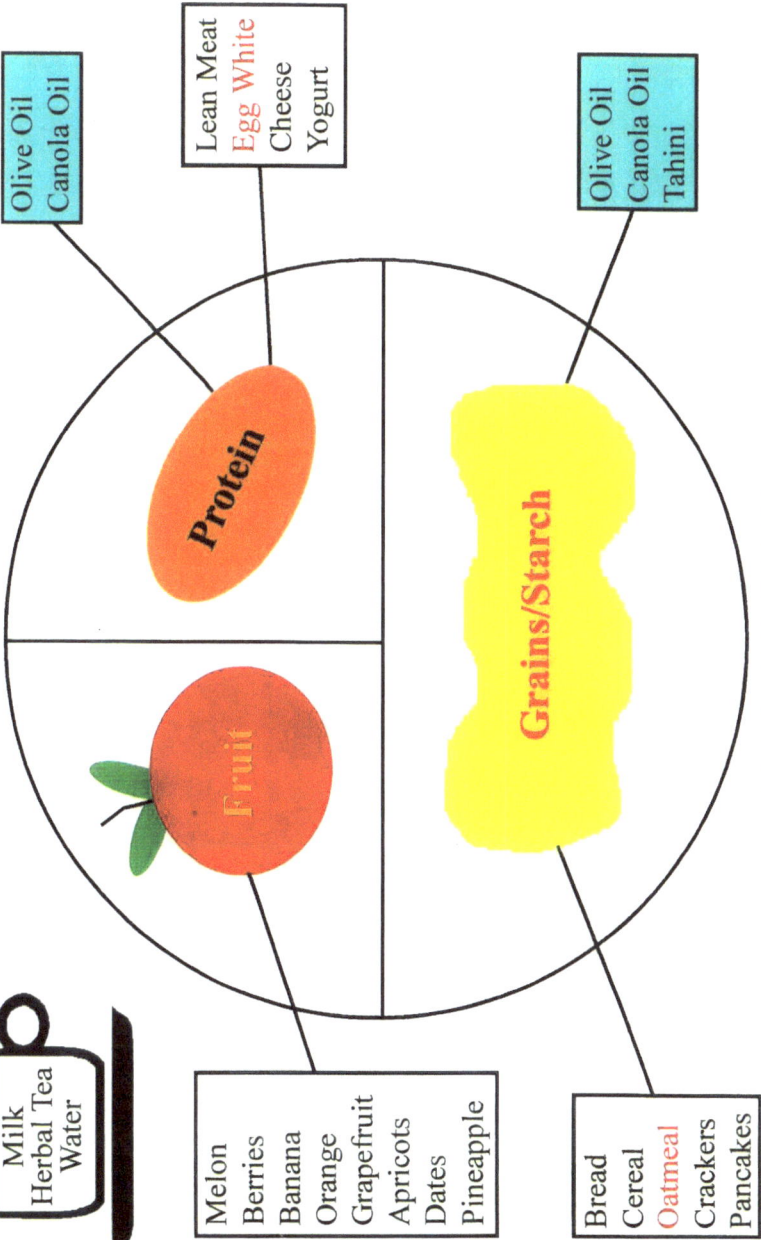

Nicholas H.E. Mezitis, M.D., ©1996

Fig. 7.1

43

Fig. 7.2

LUNCH / DINNER

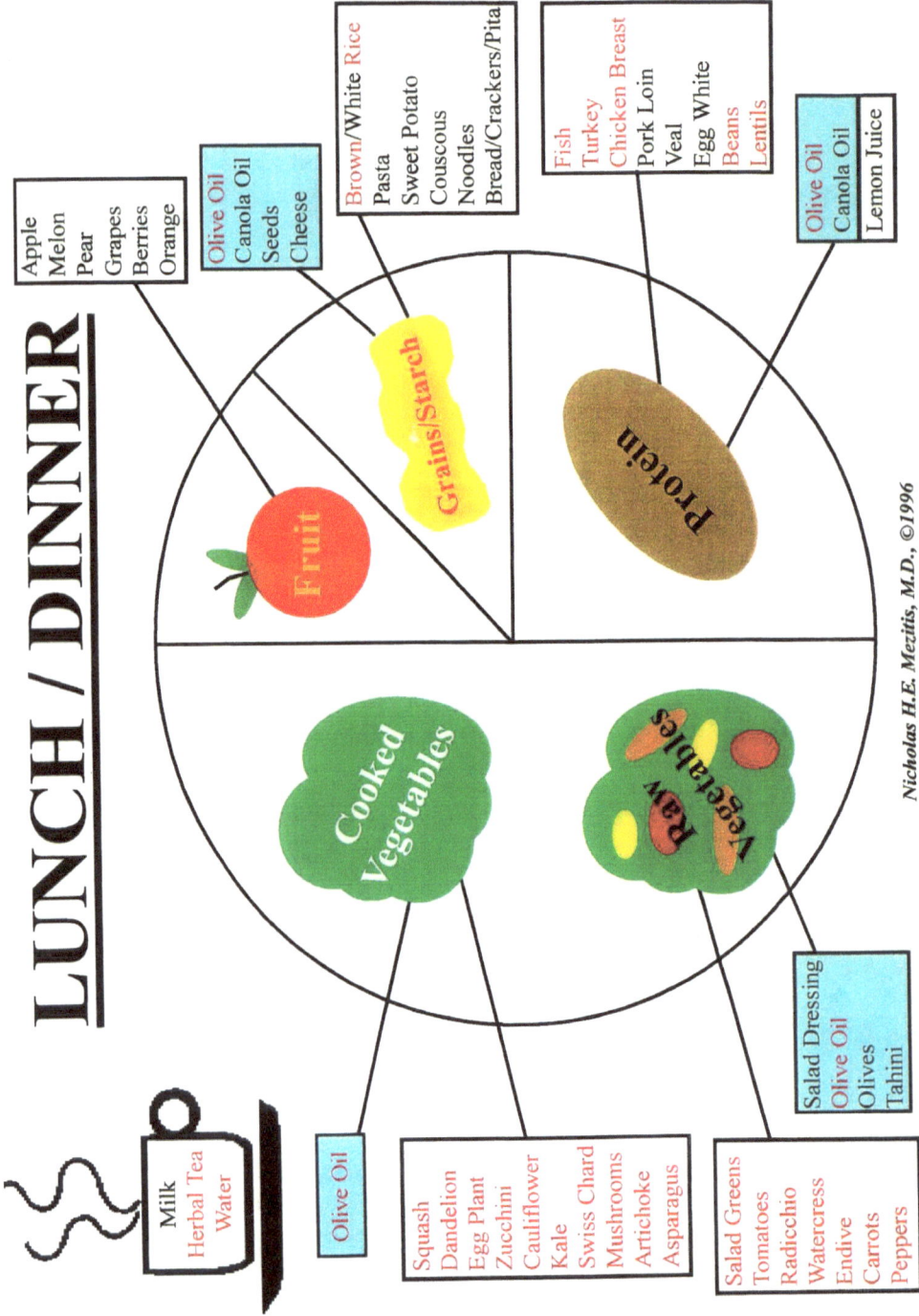

Milk
Herbal Tea
Water

Apple
Melon
Pear
Grapes
Berries
Orange

Olive Oil
Canola Oil
Seeds
Cheese

Brown/White Rice
Pasta
Sweet Potato
Couscous
Noodles
Bread/Crackers/Pita

Fish
Turkey
Chicken Breast
Pork Loin
Veal
Egg White
Beans
Lentils

Olive Oil
Canola Oil
Lemon Juice

Fruit

Grains/Starch

Protein

Cooked Vegetables

Raw Vegetables

Olive Oil

Squash
Dandelion
Egg Plant
Zucchini
Cauliflower
Kale
Swiss Chard
Mushrooms
Artichoke
Asparagus

Salad Greens
Tomatoes
Radicchio
Watercress
Endive
Carrots
Peppers

Salad Dressing
Olive Oil
Olives
Tahini

Nicholas H.E. Mezitis, M.D., ©1996

'Meals for Success'

Breakfast

Sample meals based on my plate models:

Consider honey for your yogurt.

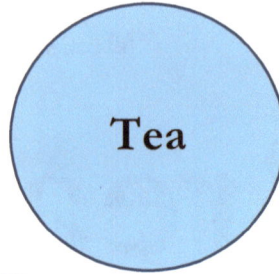

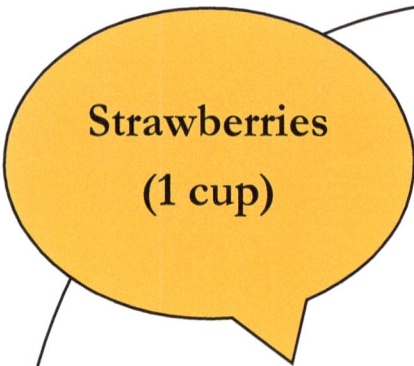

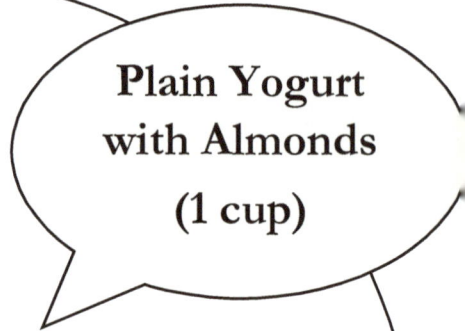

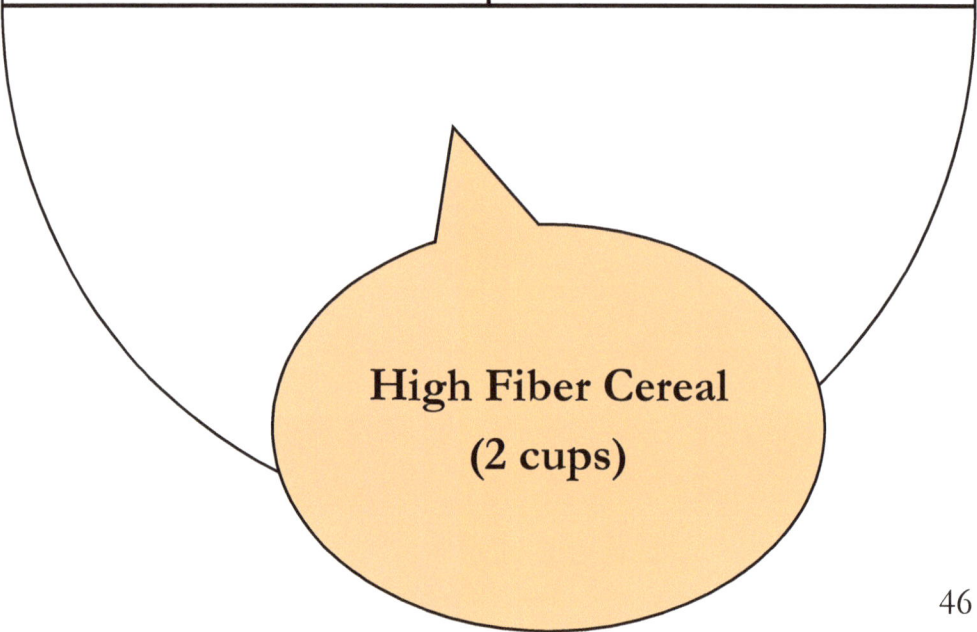

Tea

Strawberries
(1 cup)

Plain Yogurt
with Almonds
(1 cup)

High Fiber Cereal
(2 cups)

Consider almond butter or peanut butter for your toast.

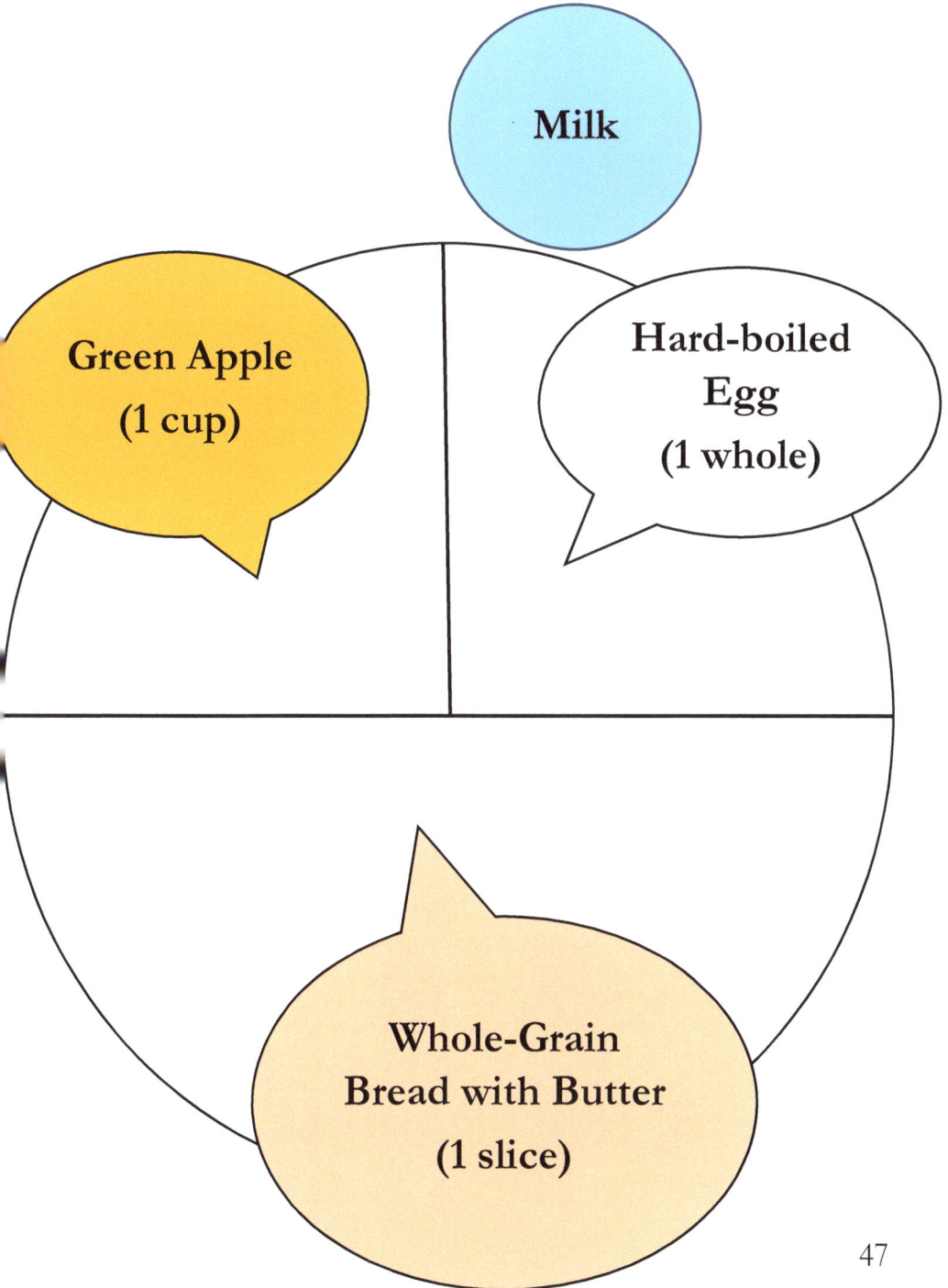

Milk

Green Apple
(1 cup)

Hard-boiled
Egg
(1 whole)

Whole-Grain
Bread with Butter
(1 slice)

Consider milk, honey, and cinnamon for your oatmeal.

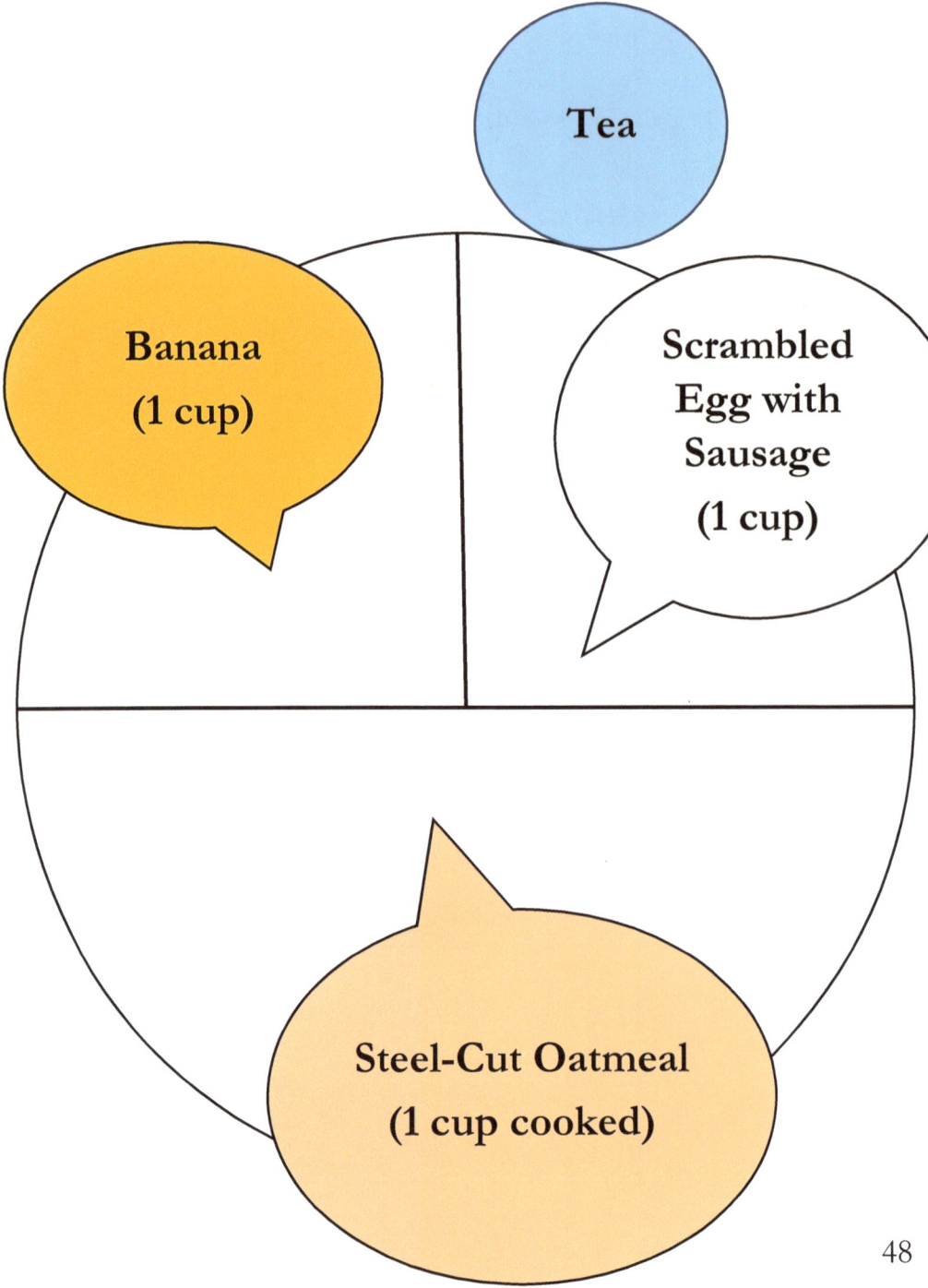

Tea

Banana
(1 cup)

Scrambled
Egg with
Sausage
(1 cup)

Steel-Cut Oatmeal
(1 cup cooked)

Make your own plate…

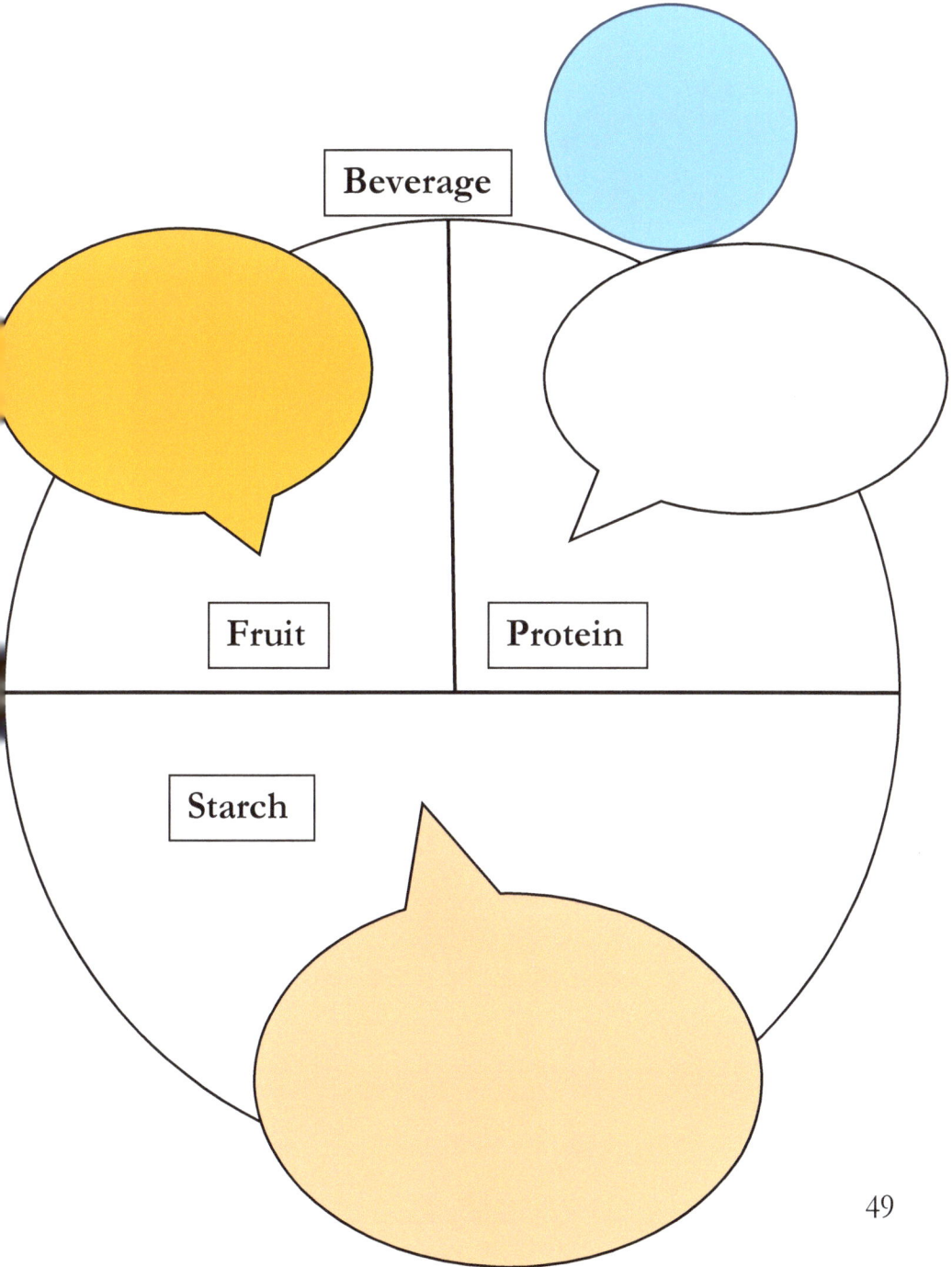

Beverage

Fruit

Protein

Starch

49

'Meals for Success'

Lunch & Dinner

Sample meals based on my plate models:

Consider Olives or Olive/Canola oil based dressings for salads.

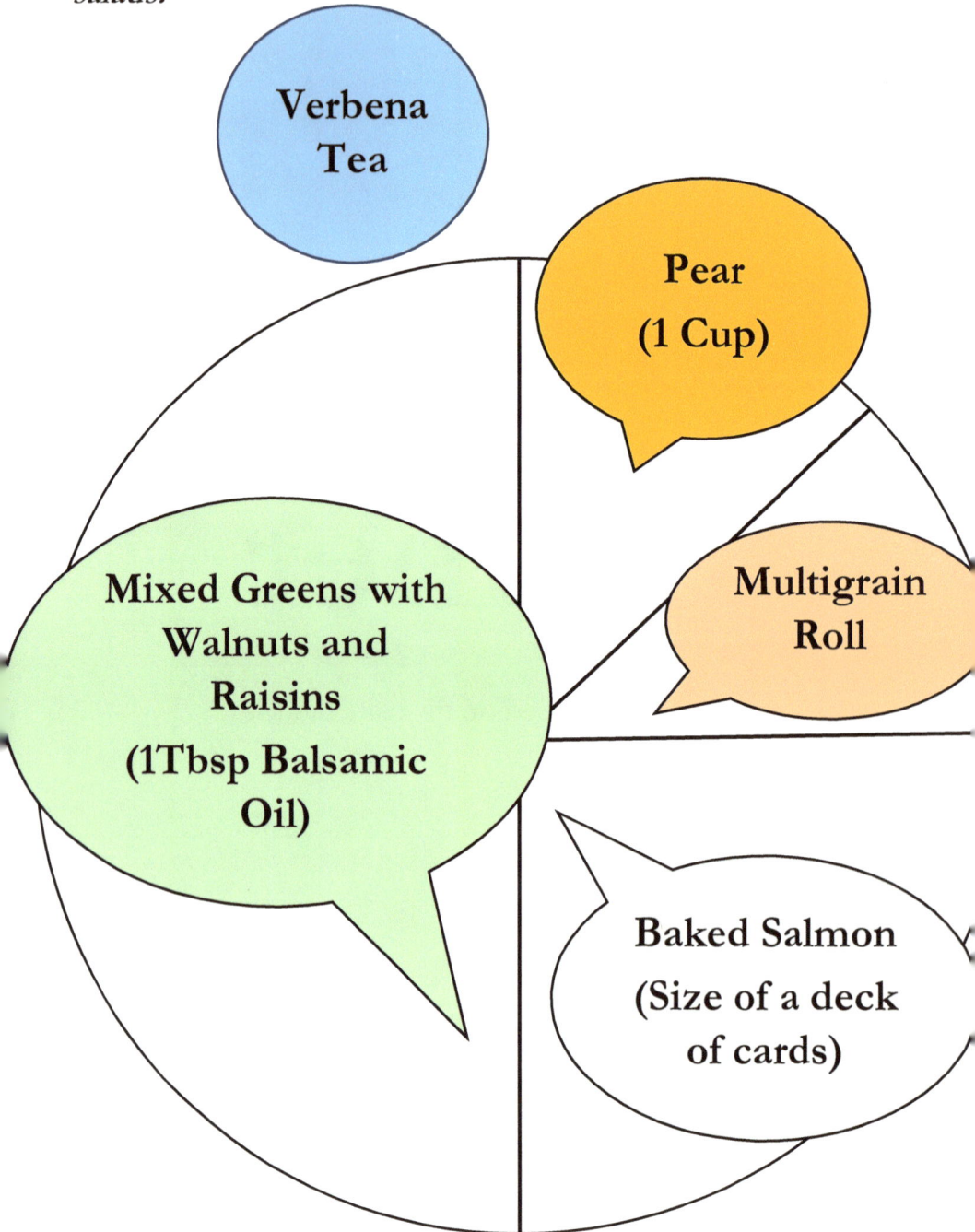

Verbena Tea

Pear (1 Cup)

Multigrain Roll

Mixed Greens with Walnuts and Raisins (1Tbsp Balsamic Oil)

Baked Salmon (Size of a deck of cards)

Consider Olives or Olive/Canola oil based dressings for vegetables.

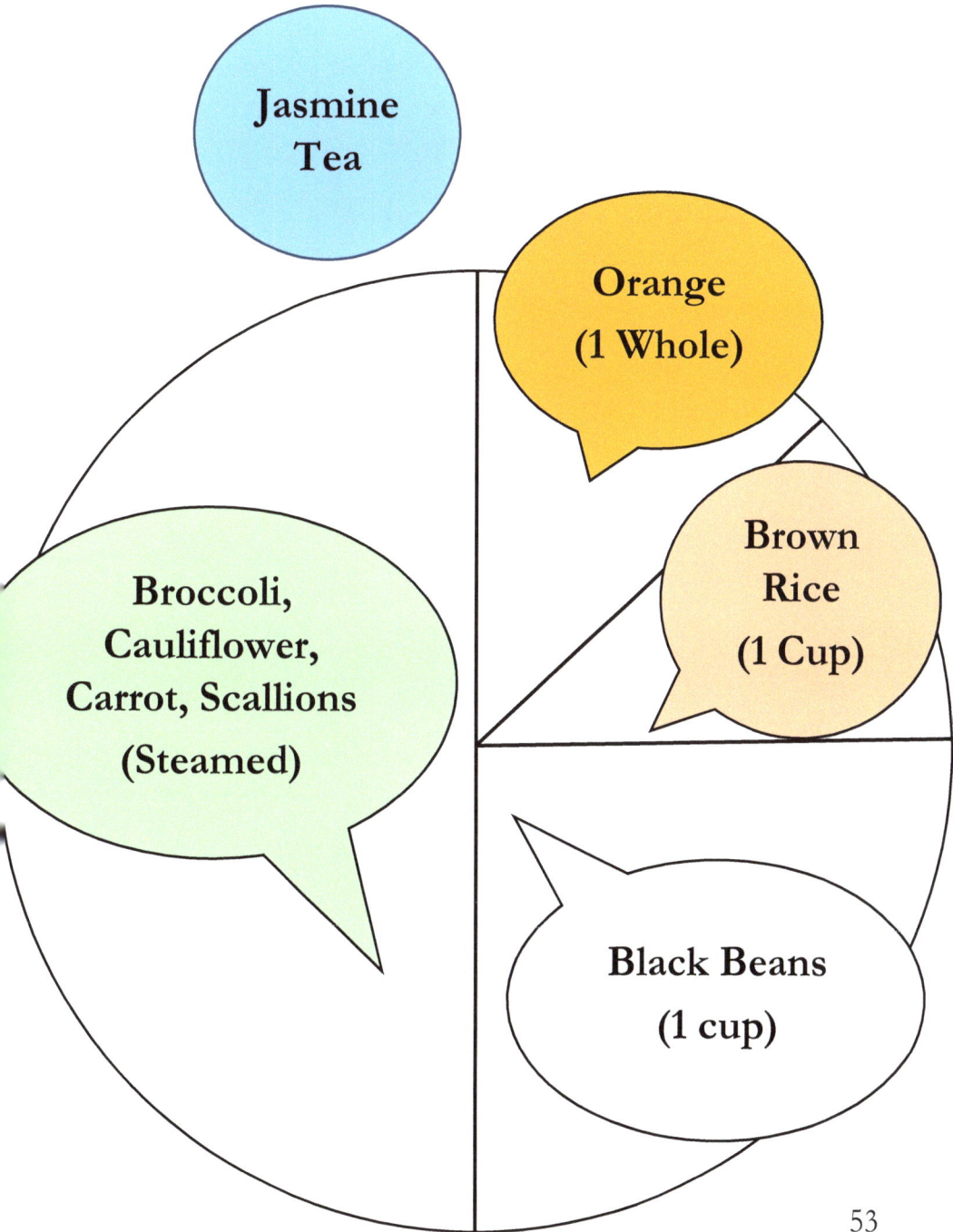

Jasmine Tea

Orange (1 Whole)

Brown Rice (1 Cup)

Broccoli, Cauliflower, Carrot, Scallions (Steamed)

Black Beans (1 cup)

Consider Olives or Olive/Canola oil based dressings for salads.

Pepper-mint Tea

Melon (1 Cup)

Orzo (1 Cup)

Tomato, Cucumber, Pepper, Onion

Lima Beans Goat Cheese

Consider a carrot or tahini dressing for the vegetables.

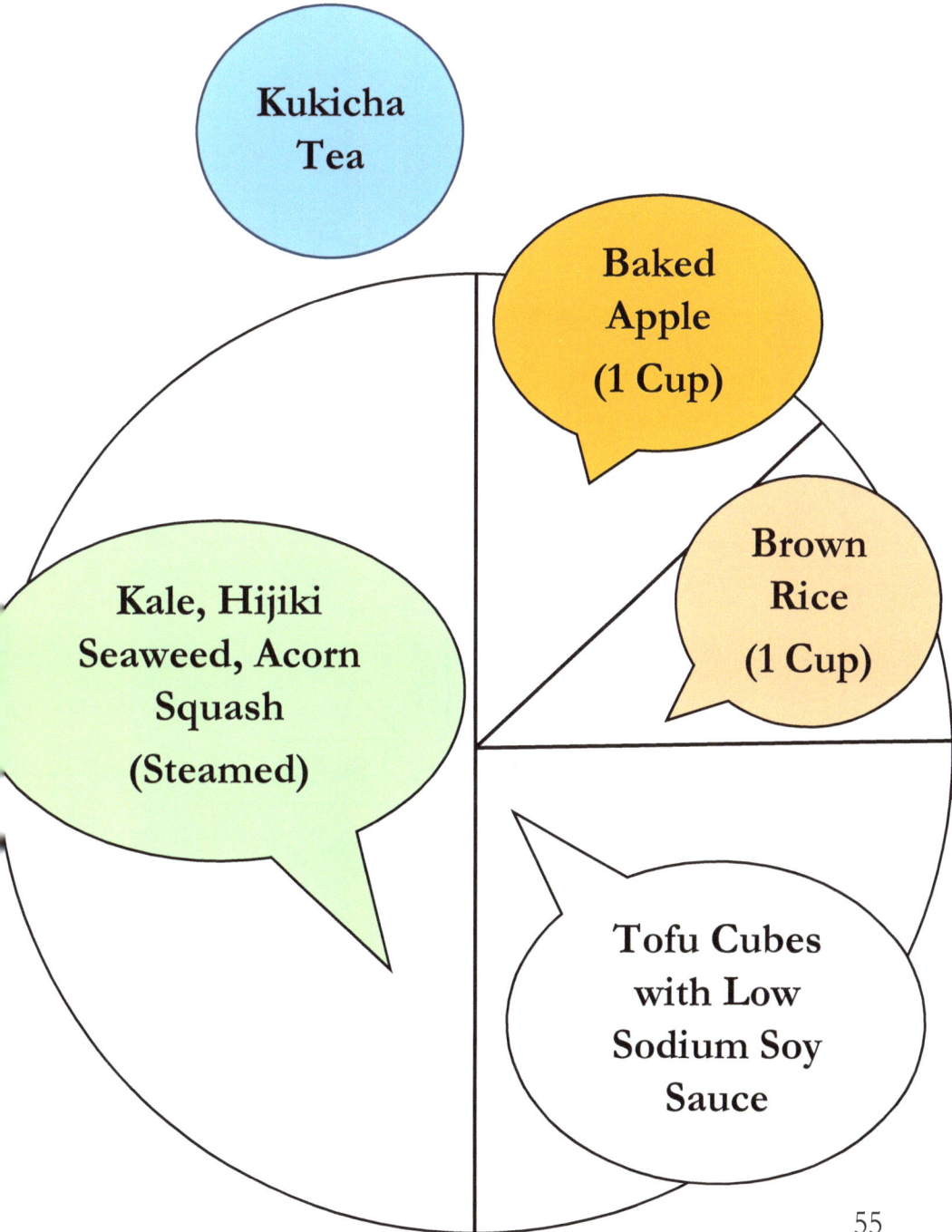

Kukicha Tea

Baked Apple (1 Cup)

Brown Rice (1 Cup)

Kale, Hijiki Seaweed, Acorn Squash (Steamed)

Tofu Cubes with Low Sodium Soy Sauce

55

Make your own plate…

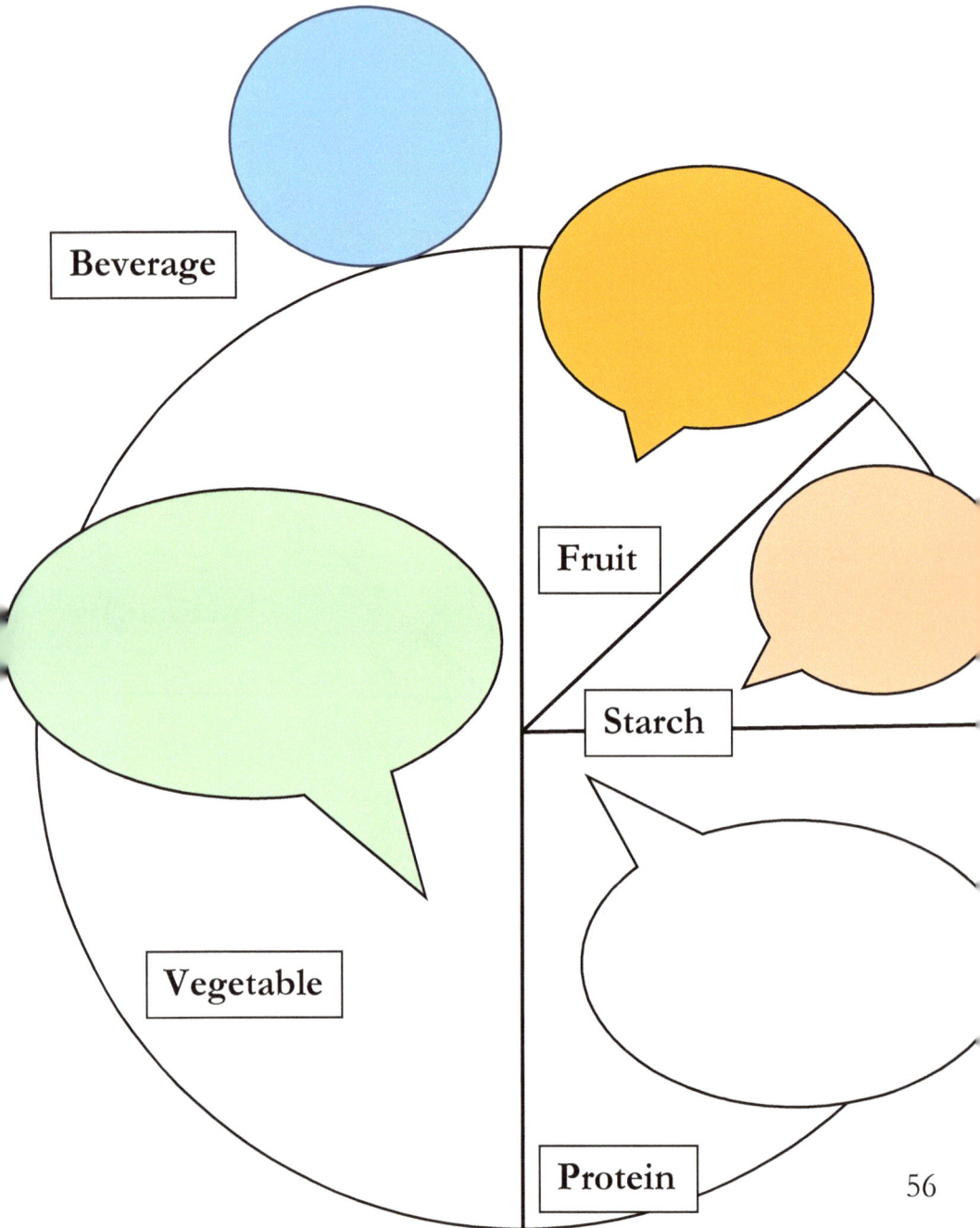

Beverage

Fruit

Starch

Vegetable

Protein

56

8

THE MEAL
"Slow food"

The M.D., the R.D., and the Chef – 'The team'

The meal served is the product of team planning and preparation. Many factors are taken into account, by us and by others, whether we realize it or not. Certainly, cultural influences and individual preferences define what comes to our plate. Health concerns and financial considerations also play an important role in making these decisions. The objective, of course, is to have a tasty, nutritious meal that will be a pleasurable experience for all.

The concept of utilizing the resources of a team of professionals is important in our multiethnic society, where food choices are varied and plentiful. As we mentioned in previous chapters, the body does not come with an instruction manual and left to our own devices it is very likely that our choices may not meet our long-term health objectives.

We have many opportunities to fall short of extracting maximum benefit from our meal. To begin with, the proportions of protein, fat, and carbohydrate may be inappropriate. Food sources for valuable vitamins and minerals may have been omitted. Fluid choices and quantities may have not been considered. The cooking procedure may have degraded vital nutrients and transformed others to damaging chemicals. Pleasing flavors may have been sacrificed in selecting foods that are not fresh and seasonal, forcing us to resort to salt and fatty dressings for the meal. Certainly, the quantities of food on the plate may be excessive. Finally, the timing of the meal may be spurious rather than consistent and the amount of time we allow for its enjoyment may be inadequate.

These important issues highlight the need to develop a plan for the meal. The resources of a nutrition team can be valuable for this purpose. The *physician* develops a nutrition prescription, taking into consideration our health status and the *dietitian* translates this recommendation into food choices and a meal outline. The *chef* provides recipes or prepares the meals highlighting the maxim 'nutritious can be delicious'.

The Dining Experience – 'Easy does it'
Food is meant to be enjoyed in a relaxed, communal setting. Dining is an opportunity to leave the stress of work and daily affairs aside and to reflect on the privilege of a full plate and of health and happiness. The company of family and friends should serve to further relax the mind and to permit digestion to proceed smoothly, without the undue intrusion of stress hormones countermanding the constructive effects of insulin (see Chapter 3).

Obviously, such an experience requires a time allowance, no different than an exercise session or a music lesson would. The mind needs a few minutes to relax. Closing the eyes for a few minutes before the meal sets the stage. Breathing enters a slow, deliberate rhythm. Muscle tension is relieved. The eyes can then appreciate the surroundings and the meal presentation. The awareness of food aromas is heightened. Digestive juices flow in anticipation of dining. When the meal is served, chewing proceeds slowly and deliberately. The meal is paced with conversation and ends with reflection on the foods consumed.

Remember, the meal is a profound event, which provides us the unique opportunity to participate in defining the makeup of our body. Genetics notwithstanding, we are in position to make the dietary choices that will improve your body composition and promote health ('You are what you eat', see Chapter 3). To abbreviate this wonderful experience, in stressful surroundings, relegating food choices and preparation to unknown parties is not a 'fast food' event. It is the equivalent of slowly starving our body of vital nutrients, until it can no longer sustain health.

Food Portions – 'Quality not quantity'

I frequently remind my patients that entrees in most restaurants in the United States can comfortably feed two people. It surprises us, when we are served a well-presented, tasty and rather small portion in an expensive restaurant. This meal, however, is usually the product of careful planning by a nutritionist and the chef. The nutritionist plans menus with an eye to calorie content and nutrient proportions. The chef selects quality ingredients and focuses on extracting flavor with skillful meal preparation, while preparing a presentation that delights the eye.

For all intents and purposes, a few simple guidelines will help you avoid excess in your food portions:

At home, serve your meal cafeteria-style in the food preparation area and avoid returning for second helpings.

In a restaurant, ask for a second plate to divide your entrée. The portion remaining can be shared or it can be packaged to be enjoyed as a meal at home.

Always plan to be 'a little hungry' when you leave the table.

Meal Timing – 'A nine – to – five schedule'

"How would you like an eighteen-wheeler to pull up at your business at 9:30 PM and unload the delivery you expected at 11:00 AM?" I asked the patient. It would be a messy experience. Boxes would flood the ramps. The janitor and security staff, hastily recruited to assist the few remaining business staff members in making space for storage inside the building, would cram boxes in hallways and office areas. Morning would bring fresh excitement, as regularly scheduled deliveries would add more packages, just as the harried staff is confronting the previous evening's events. Obviously, the day's activities would proceed with the usual intense rhythm, further exacerbating tensions. Stress would be rampant and tempers would run short. "Unthinkable," my patient responded.

This is exactly the experience we seek to avoid for our metabolism. Home economics at the cellular level works on a circadian light-dark cycle. The body 'wakes up' at dawn, whether we decide to leave our bed or not. It 'goes to bed' with sunset, regardless of whether we are preparing for a night on the town. Sensitive hormonal rhythms attest to this fact (see Chapter 3) and the digestive processes follow suit. To force the frequently sleep-deprived body to accept food deliveries at odd hours of the night and to whip it into submission with stimulants such as coffee or alcohol is definitely not conducive to a productive long-term relationship.

Experiments have shown that the body disposes of a meal most easily in the morning. The same amount of food consumed at lunchtime will take twice as long to manage. As a late dinner, the standard meal mentioned will keep the body's resources mobilized all night to secure disposal. For our purposes, I recommend a hearty breakfast, followed by a light lunch, and a dinner to be completed no later than 8:00 PM. Should the schedule call for late evening socializing, one can always resort to a light snack, if a meal is planned as part of the activities.

Conventional Meal Timing

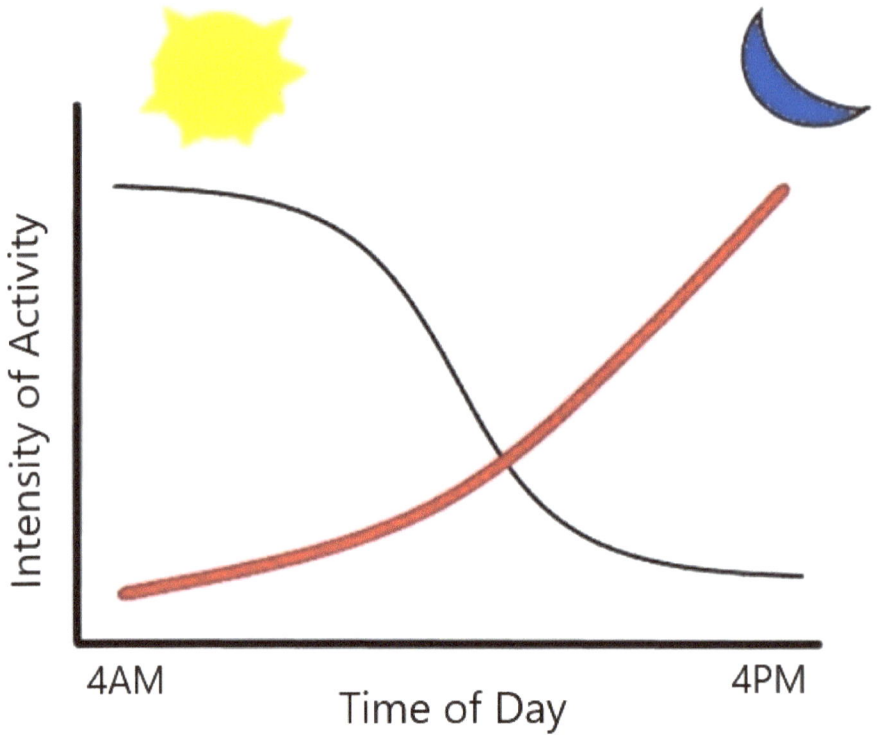

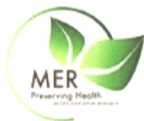

Desirable Meal Timing

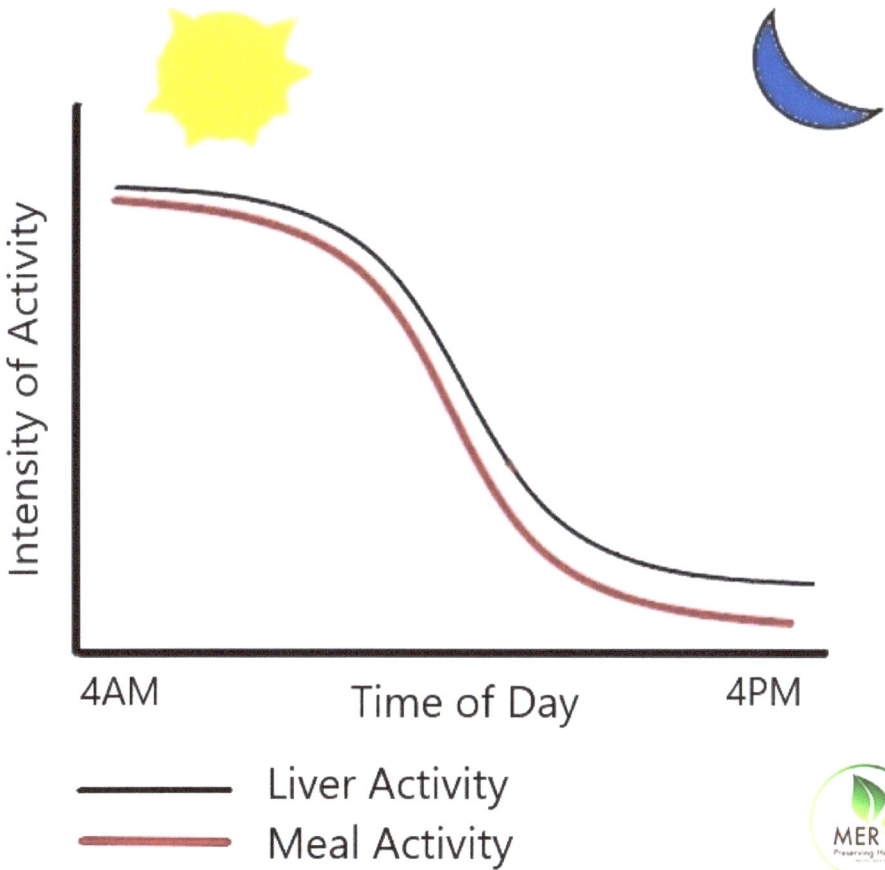

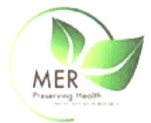

9

FOOD IS YOUR MEDICINE
"Postponing graduation"

Insulin Resistance – 'Is anyone home?'
In Greek mythology, a tormented soul thirsts in the middle of a beautiful lake. Every time he lowers his head to drink, the water level drops ever so slightly, always remaining at the level of his lower lip. Maintaining fuel economy in our bodies has become increasingly difficult in the past half-century. Just as one would expect that plentiful harvests and limited demands for physical exertion should have secured for us a sunny "Garden of Eden" experience on earth, clouds have appeared.

The body's fuel sensor, the 'beta cell', whose function we described in Chapter 3, produces the insulin we need to make use of the food we consume. Interestingly, eating less and exercising more makes the beta cell happy. Less food and certainly less carbohydrate means less stimulation to produce and release insulin. More exercise makes the body's tissues more receptive to the effects of insulin and means we get 'more mileage' for less insulin produced. Fuel economy doesn't get better than this.

Unfortunately, the apple the serpent offered in our version of events is the false promise that physical inactivity is bliss. Cars, elevators, electrical appliances, the telephone and the Internet have all offered us the opportunity to rule an empire with our fingers doing most of the walking. The result was unanticipated: insulin resistance.

Sensitivity to insulin's action and insulin resistance are two faces of the same coin. The less sensitive we become to insulin's message as it binds to our tissue receptors, the more resistant we are. The beta cell puts up a good show to be sure. It pumps out more and more insulin at every meal trying to keep the situation under control and most of the time it succeeds in clearing the foods from the blood stream and maintaining harmony in our 'metabolic melody' (see Chapter 3). Large amounts of insulin in circulation come at a price however. Inflation in the body's fuel economy is no less desirable than on Wall Street and the consequences can be dire. Insulin is a potent appetite stimulant and a powerful growth hormone. It can make the body load up on fat and water and drive up its blood pressure. It may also ruin the tubing that serves circulation by promoting overgrowth of its lining; a process we know as arteriosclerosis.

The results of this drama unfolding are witnessed everywhere, surrounded as we are by an overweight population unable to control its appetite. Emergency rooms are filled with patients suffering from heart attacks and strokes. Billions of dollars flow to the pharmaceutical industry for medication to lower blood pressure, cholesterol levels, and to drive water from the body. Adding insult to injury, a massively expensive research effort is underway searching for the Holy Grail, the 'obesity cure'.

For most people however, the 'warm up' skits are destined to end, as the beta cell strains to keep up with an unfamiliar lifestyle and delivers the spirit. Rising insulin levels no longer suffice to meet the excessive requirements. Sugar and other vital nutrients back up in the system, unable to be utilized efficiently. Rising glucose levels in the blood swiftly exceed the thresholds defined as 'normal' and diabetes mellitus makes its unwelcome appearance.

This unpleasant sequence of events is becoming all too familiar in our population. Over 650,000 people develop diabetes every year, many of them children. The overwhelming majority still produces insulin, but their production is inadequate for their lifestyle of choice. An estimated 16 million individuals in the United States have this problem and the results are devastating. Circulating in the blood vessels, a defective fuel mix rich in sugar and triglycerides ruins their lining and leads to their gradual destruction. In the eyes it means blindness, in the kidneys renal failure, in the feet gangrene, in the genitals impotence and the list goes on. Premature aging and untimely death are the result.

Exercise – 'Use it or lose it'
Restoring the body to its balance and maintaining health requires a regular program of exercise. This can be as simple as walking and stretching or as ambitious as we wish, but it must be consistent. The rewards are great, since experiments confirm that utilization of nutrients such as glucose improves rapidly following physical activity and the benefits are sustained for the entire day. I

recommend a pedometer to guide you in your daily activity. The objective would be a minimum of 10,000 steps a day.

Food as Medicine

Keeping our nutrition 'label' (see Chapter 5) in mind is key in avoiding the pitfalls described earlier. Food can nourish the body, but it can also express a function in protecting from toxins and restoring balance. Peroxide radicals formed by metabolic processes may harm the tissues. Antioxidants in our foods can neutralize their effects. Acids form as the result of body functions. Alkaline-rich food choices can maintain the body's acid-base (pH) balance. Foods rich in simple carbohydrates can release glucose in excessive amounts to the blood stream. Other food choices such as legumes/beans containing antinutrients can delay the digestion of these carbohydrates and postpone the absorption of glucose, easing the burden on the beta cell.

The food supply is full of such valuable items, which when properly selected and combined can keep us healthy and vigorous for many years to come. Graduation from this life can be comfortably postponed.

10

PARTING WORDS
"The Center Line"

"So," the young woman said, leaning slightly towards my desk and glancing at the overweight lady sitting next to her, who had been doing much of the talking. "We will be getting a diet for my mother's blood pressure …?" "No," I replied. "We will be discussing a diet for your mother and your family, not for her blood pressure. You see, the plan we provide will guide you in preparing flavorful, balanced meals that your entire family can enjoy. Your mother's blood pressure will benefit, but more importantly, her children and grandchildren may avoid similar problems in the future. After all, her medical history is a glimpse into the crystal ball for the family members…"

This book has hopefully served to highlight that there is no 'problem food' and there is no 'healthy food'. The issues to be addressed, as we plan our meal, relate to food quality and quantity. If we accept that our 'food is our medicine', then we have to behave accordingly. The same medicine can heal or poison, depending on its provenance and the amount consumed. We don't usually swallow extra pills on our prescribed antibiotic because 'we're bored' or because 'they taste good'. We shouldn't expect to spend the better part of the day munching on snacks and slurping beverages, because we find the experience comforting.

Ideally, any food we enjoy will find an opportunity to make its appearance on our meal plate over the course of a week. For some food items that have low nutritional value and a lengthy list of additives on the label, we make it a rare occurrence. These rare and fleeting moments of pleasure should not be our focus as we plan the meal. *The Plate with protein, fat, and carbohydrate in colorful balance should be dominating in our mind's eye as we sit at the table.*

Seasonal vegetables, fresh, steamed or braised occupy half the Plate. Fish, meat, beans, poultry or an occasional egg find themselves in their niche. Bread, potatoes, rice or pasta are quite limited in their representation, but they are present. Fat, usually in the form of vegetable oils, may find its place as a flavorful companion to any one of the groupings mentioned. Its appearance is restricted, but it wouldn't be a party without it. Fresh fruits are nature's dessert and they're certainly invited to the meal, in moderation. The beverage, an herbal tea or cool water, is readily available to slake thirst and maintain our fluid reserves.

Our objective is to develop a dietary lifestyle that becomes second nature for us. A critical element, such as vegetables or protein, missing from the Plate would be reason to postpone dining. The body appreciates protein, fat and carbohydrate in all their variety and expects them to make a joint appearance as a 'mixed meal'. Using protein for fuel, because carbohydrate is unavailable, or not having a timely delivery of amino acids, vital to building tissue, is not in its concept of fuel economy. As such, the concept of our

Meal Plate supersedes the 'wheels' and 'pyramids' of nutrition lore, since **we expect balance at every meal with meals timed in harmony with the body's sleep-wake cycle**, not merely a satisfactory tally of daily portions, no matter what their distribution and timing.

There is a wealth of colorful and insightful literature in bookstores relating to food choices and food preparation. Diet seminars and cooking classes are offered in abundance. It is my sincere hope that your **Blueprint for Healthy Eating** will be a useful guide and faithful companion as you enjoy the well-deserved pleasures of constructing your favorite meals.

11
APPENDIX
"Tables and Resources"

Table A.1: Dietary Antioxidants (1)

Antioxidant Team	Good Food Sources	Recommended Dietary Allowance (adult)	Food Equivalent
Vitamin C (Ascorbic Acid)	Citrus fruits and juices, tomatoes, melon, peppers, strawberries.	Males: 60 mg Females: 60 mg	This is equivalent to the amount found in one medium orange, or 1/2 cup of broccoli.
Vitamin E	Almonds, avocado, brown rice, dry beans, egg yolks, green leafy vegetables, milk, rolled oats.	Males: 10 mg Females: 8 mg	This is equivalent to the amount found in 1.5 oz of almonds, or 1/2 cup wheat germ.
Beta-carotene and the Carotenoids	Apricots, cantaloupe, carrots, squash, spinach, sweet potatoes.	Not established	
Soy Isoflavones and the Bioflavonoids	Soybeans and products, blueberries, purple grapes.	Not established	
Coenzyme Q10 and the Ubiquinones	Liver, peanuts, sardines.	Not established	
Selenium	Egg yolks, tuna, seafood, liver, whole grains, plants grown in selenium rich soil.	Males: 70 mcg Females: 55 mcg	This is equivalent to the amount found in 6 oz of chicken, or 2 cups of brown rice.

References: Dietary Antioxidants

Rock CL, Jacob RA, Bowen PE. Update on the biological characteristics of antioxidant micronutrients: vitamin C, Vitamin E, and the carotenoids. *Journal of the American Dietetic Association.* 1996; 96(7) 693-702.

Monsen ER. Dietary reference intakes for antioxidant nutrients: vitamin C, vitamin E, selenium and carotenoids. *Journal of the American Dietetic Association.* 2000; 100(6): 637-40.

Table A.2: Decoding Food Labels (1)

Claim	Meaning
Calorie-free	One serving contains fewer than 5 calories per serving
Cholesterol-free	One serving contains less than 2 mg of cholesterol, and/or less than or equal to 2 g of saturated fat
Excellent Source	One serving contains 20%, or more of the daily value for a particular nutrient
Extra Lean (seafood, game, poultry, meat)	One Serving (3 oz) contains less than 5 g fat, 2 g saturated fat, and 95 mg cholesterol
Fat Free	One serving contains less than 0.5 g of fat
Free	One serving contains a negligible amount (not none at all)
Good Source	One serving contains 10-19% of the daily value for a particular nutrient
Healthy	One serving is low in fat and saturated fat, contains at least 10% of the Daily Value for Vitamins A and C, calcium, fiber, iron, and protein, and contains 480 mg, or less sodium

Table A.3: Decoding Food Labels (2)

High	One serving contains 20%, or more of the daily value for a particular nutrient
Lean (seafood, game, poultry, meat)	One serving (3 oz) contains less than 10 g fat, no more than 4.5 g saturated fat, and less than 95 mg cholesterol
Light ("lite")	The modified product contains 1/3 of the calories, 50% less sodium, or 50% less fat than the standard product
Low Calorie	One serving contains less than, or equal to 40 calories
Low Cholesterol	One serving contains less than, or equal to 20 mg of cholesterol
Low Fat ("lowfat")	One serving contains less than, or equal to 3 g of fat
Low Saturated Fat	One serving contains less than, or equal to 1 g of saturated fat
More	One serving contains at least 10%, or more of the Daily Value of a specified nutrient
Reduced	One serving of contains at least 25% less calories, fat, saturated fat, cholesterol, or sodium than one serving of the standard product

Table A.4: Decoding Food Labels (3)

Sugar-free	One serving contains less than 0.5 g sugar
Sodium-free	One serving contains less than 5 mg sodium

Table A.5: Cuisine Choices (1)

Cuisine	Healthier Choices	"Sometimes" Foods
"American"	Vegetable soup	Cream soup
	Vinaigrette dressings	Creamy dressings
	Tossed salad (side dressing)	Mayonnaise based salad
	"Lean" hamburger	Cheese/bacon hamburger
	Turkey/chicken sandwich	Corned beef/pastrami sand.
	Baked potato (plain)	Home fries/French fries
Chinese	Wonton/hot-n-sour soup	Egg drop soup
	Steamed vegetable dumplings	Fried dumplings/egg rolls
	Chicken w/ vegetables	General Tso's
	Beef w/ vegetables	Lo Mein
	Moo shu	Sesame chicken
	Sauteed shrimp w/vegetables	Chow fun
	White/brown rice	Fried rice
	Sweet and sour sauces	Sesame/peanut sauces

Table A.6: Cuisine Choices (2)

Cuisine	Healthier Choices	"Sometimes" Foods
Greek (Middle-Eastern)	Fresh salad (side dressing) Pita bread Steamed mussels/calamari Grilled kebabs Fresh fish	Spanakopita Falafel (fried) Fried calamari Pastitsio (cream casserole) Baklava
Indian	Curried vegetables Okra/spinach Dal (bean puree) Tandoori dishes Basmati rice	Coconut based sauces Lamb dishes Cream sauces
Italian	Minestrone soup Pasta primavera Pasta Marinara/Neapolitan Grilled chicken/fish Thin crust pizza Italian ices	Garlic bread Pasta alla vodka Fettuccini Alfredo Parmesan/Lasagna dishes Italian sausages Cannoli/Napoleon

Table A.7: Cuisine Choices (3)

Cuisine	Healthier Choices	"Sometimes" Foods
Japanese	Miso soup Edamame (soy beans) Sushi/sashimi	Tempura Fried dishes
Mexican (Tex-Mex)	Gazpacho Tortilla chips w/salsa Grilled Fajitas Vegetable filled tortillas	Nachos Fried tortillas/tacos Taco salad Refried beans

Table A.8: Food Handling (1)

Food Item	Raw Handling Tips	Safe Cooking Temperatures (Internal)	How to take the temp/when is it done?	Refrigeration Limit: Keeps up to…	Storage Suggestions
Beef, Lamb, Veal: -Ground Items -Roasts/Steaks (rare-well)	Never defrost on the kitchen counter.	160 F 145-170 F	Insert thermometer into center of the thickest part.	3-4 days	Keep packages of raw meat, poultry and fish wrapped separately. Store them on the lowest shelf--it is usually the coldest. Also, storing them there may prevent juices from dripping on other foods.
Poultry: -Ground Items -Whole Bird -Boneless Breasts and Roasts -Thighs, Wings, Drumsticks -Duck, Goose	Freeze these foods immediately if raw products are not to be used within a few days.	165 F 180 F 170 F 180 F 180 F	For the whole bird: insert thermometer into the inner thigh, near the breast, but do not touch the bone.	3-4 days	
Pork: -All Cuts (medium-well) -Fresh, Raw Ham -Fully Cooked Ham (reheat)	Use plastic cutting boards. Marinate inside of the refrigerator, not on the counter.	160-170 F 180 F 140 F	Insert thermometer into the thickest part.	3-4 days (cooked)	
Fish			Cook until opaque and flakes easily with a fork.	2 days (cooked)	

Table A.9: Food Handling (2)

Food Item	Raw Handling Tips	Safe Cooking Temperatures (Internal)	How to take the temp/when is it done?	Refrigeration Limit: Keeps up to...	Storage Suggestions
Egg Dishes, Casseroles: Raw eggs:	If bought pre-packaged, use by sell-date.	160 F	Insert into the thickest area of the dish.	3 days 3 weeks (in shell)	
Leftovers	Do not serve with the same utensils used for food preparation.	165 F	Insert into the thickest area of the dish	3-5 days	Store in air-tight containers. Divide large amounts into small containers.
Vegetables: -Raw -Cooked	Wash thoroughly.			1 Week 3-4 Days	Blanch vegetables before freezing.
Grains: -Cooked Pasta -Cooked Rice -Stuffing				3-5 Days 1 Week 1-2 Days	

Table A.10: Dietary Reference Intake (1)

Dietary Reference Intake (DRI): A term designated for nutrient recommendations in the United States and Canada. DRIs are the most recent set of dietary recommendations established by the Food and Nutrition Board of the Institute of Medicine, 1997-2001.

Vitamins and Minerals	RDA/AI for Adult Males	RDA/AI for Non-Pregnant/Non-Lactating Adult Females	Adult UL1 (maximum level that is likely to pose no risk of adverse effects)	Sample Food Choices
Biotin	30 mg	30 mg	ND²	Rolled oats Peanut butter
Calcium	1,000 mg (ages 19-50) 1,200 mg (ages 51+)	1,000 mg (ages 19-50) 1,200 mg (ages 51+)	2,500 mg	Skim milk Tofu
Choline	550 mg	425 mg	3,500 mg	Skim Milk Egg
Chromium	35 micrograms (ages 19-50) 30 micrograms (ages >50)	25 micrograms (ages 19-50) 20 micrograms (ages >50)	ND²	Some cereals Meats, poultry, fish
Copper	900 micrograms	900 micrograms	10,000 micrograms (10 mg)	Nuts Seeds
Fluoride	4 mg	3 mg	10 mg	Drinking water Marine Fish
Folate	400 micrograms	400 micrograms	1,000 micrograms	Enriched cereal Spinach
Iodine	150 micrograms	150 micrograms	1,100 micrograms	Salt, iodized Shrimp
Iron	8 mg	18 mg (age 19-50) 8 mg (age 50 and up)	45 mg	Ground Beef, lean Poultry

Table A.11: Dietary Reference Intake (2)

Vitamins and Minerals	RDA/AI for Adult Males	RDA/AI for Non-Pregnant/Non-Lactating Adult Females	Adult UL1 (maximum level that is likely to pose no risk of adverse effects)	Sample Food Choices
Magnesium	400 mg (ages 19-30) 420 mg (ages 31+)	310 mg (ages 19-30) 320 mg (ages 31+)	350 mg	Nuts Green leafy vegetables
Niacin	16 mg	14 mg	35 mg	Fish Fortified grains
Pantothenic Acid	5 mg	5 mg	ND[2]	Chicken Broccoli
Phosphorous	700 mg	700 mg	4,000 mg (ages 19-70) 3,000 mg (ages >70)	Peas Yogurt
Riboflavin	1.3 mg	1.1 mg	ND[2]	Skim milk Fortified cereals
Selenium	55 micrograms	55 micrograms	400 micrograms	Seafood Organ meats
Thiamin	1.2 mg	1.1 mg	ND[2]	Fortified grains, Breads, cereals
Vitamin A (includes provitamin A carotenoids)	*900 micrograms	700 micrograms	3,000 micrograms	Carrots Spinach
Vitamin B6 (Pyridoxine)	1.3 mg (ages 19-50) 1.7 mg (ages 51+)	1.3 mg (ages 19-50) 1.5 mg (ages 51+)	100 mg	Banana Potato
Vitamin B12	**2.4 micrograms	***2.4 micrograms	ND[2]	Beef, lean Fish
Vitamin C	90 mg	75 mg	2,000 mg	Cantaloupe Orange Juice

Notes:

<u>Recommended Dietary Allowances (RDAs)</u> In **bold type**, <u>Adequate Intakes (AIs)</u> in ordinary type. RDAs and AIs may both be used as goals for individual intake. RDAs are set to meet the needs of almost all (97 to 98 percent) individuals in a group. The AI for adults is believed to cover the needs of all individuals in the group, but lack of data prevents being able to specify with confidence the percentage of individuals covered by this intake.

[1]<u>UL</u>: The maximum level of daily nutrient intake that is likely to pose no risk of adverse effects. Unless otherwise specified, the UL represents total intake from food, water, and supplements. Due to lack of suitable data, ULs could not be established for vitamin K, thiamin, riboflavin, vitamin B12, pantothenic acid, biotin, or carotenoids. In the absence of ULs, extra caution may be warranted in consuming levels above recommended intakes.

[2]ND: Not determinable due to lack of data of adverse effects in this age group and concern of inability to handle excess amounts. Source of intake should be from food only to prevent high levels of intake.

* Given as retinal activity equivalents (RAEs). 1 RAE = 1 µgretinol, 12 µg β-carotene, 24 µg α-carotene, or 24 µg cryptoxanthin. To calculate RAEs from REs of provitamin A carotenoids in foods, divide the REs by 2. For preformed vitamin

A in foods or supplements and for provitamin A carotenoids in supplements, 1 RE = 1 RAE.

** It is recommended that adults over the age of 50 meet the RDA for vitamin B_{12} by consuming B_{12} fortified foods and/or a supplement containing B_{12}. This recommendation is made based on the finding that 10-30% of older people may malabsorb food-bound vitamin B_{12}.

*** Vitamin D in the above table is listed in the form of cholecalciferol. 1 microgram cholecalciferol = 40 IU vitamin D. The above RDIs for Vitamin D are made in the assumed absence of adequate sunlight.

Information found in the above tables was adapted from:

Dietary Reference Intakes for Calcium, Phosphorous, Magnesium, Vitamin D, and Fluoride (1997); *Dietary Reference Intakes for Thiamin, Riboflavin, Niacin, Vitamin B6, Folate, Vitamin B12, Pantothenic Acid, Biotin, and Choline* (1998); *Dietary Reference Intakes for Vitamin C, Vitamin E, Selenium, and Carotenoids* (2000); and *Dietary Reference*

Intakes for Vitamin A, Vitamin K, Arsenic, Boron, Chromium, Copper, Iodine, Iron, Manganese, Molybdenum, Nickel, Silicon, Vanadium, and Zinc (2001). These reports may be accessed via www. Copyright 2001 by The National Academies. All rights reserved.

www.ingramcontent.com/pod-product-compliance
Lightning Source LLC
Chambersburg PA
CBHW040125270326
41926CB00001B/22